Contents....

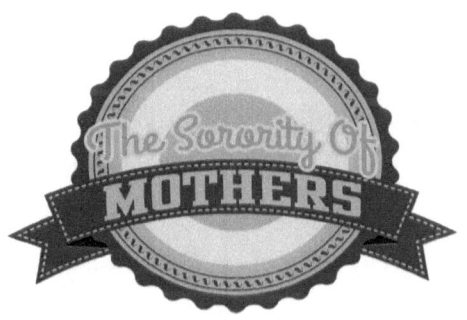

Infertility: A Growing Problem for So Many Women

When you imagine having a baby in your life you more than likely think of it as a very natural process. It may very well be something that you have envisioned and even dreamed of since a young age. For many women having children is part of the natural cycle of life and therefore something that they automatically assume will happen for them someday.

However, for a growing number of women the whole notion of getting pregnant may be much harder than you might realize. So what can you do if you happen to be one of the many women out there who struggle with fertility issues? How can you handle them and make it through a potentially challenging process? In this book we look at getting you through the emotional stages and on to practical solutions to help you fall pregnant.

Fertility Issues are the last things on anyone's mind when they first start trying for a baby. It has however, become a very unfortunate reality for so many women and it seems to be on the rise. While some women may get pregnant the very first time they try, others may struggle for months or even years with the process.

This can make for a very frustrating experience and can put a cloud over many other areas of your life. If you can identify with this experience and feel the struggle personally then you are not alone!

Many people believe that fertility issues have come about due to environmental factors. We eat far more processed foods than we used to. We breathe air that isn't as clean and generally just don't look after ourselves as good as we could.

A lot of women are waiting to have children until later in their lives and this too may contribute to the problem. Add the stress and worry of day to day life and you can see why so many women are struggling to get pregnant and have the baby they dream of.

It doesn't matter what your personal issue is, what sort of health condition or lifestyle you come with, or what personal struggles you have—the bottom line is that it can be very frustrating and stressful when you can't get pregnant as quickly or easily as you'd like.

Though many people in your own life may not understand what it feels like, there are plenty of others out there going through the exact same situation. This problem has evolved into a phenomenon and within that is the anxiety, frustration, and challenges that wanting to have a baby can bring about.

It's Time to Talk About It From a Real Point of View

This book is written from a very sympathetic and down to earth point of view to reach out, help, inform and offer real solutions to women struggling with this problem. Whether you've been trying for a month or for years, your issues with getting pregnant are very real.

There are many books available on the subject of getting pregnant, and you can get some great medical information however this book is intended to help you through every aspect of the process.

Sure your doctor can help you to uncover the medical reasons as to why you may be struggling and that's very important, but we aim to help you to come to terms with what you are feeling, help you to work through it and give you real and practical pregnancy alternatives.

Tackling the Problem

Though you may feel isolated or alone or like you are the only one struggling with getting pregnant, you will find some comfort and help in the information and ideas within these pages.

It's time to speak from a very real point of view. It's time to look at treatments that may be out there that can start from the minute that you feel frustrated. It may be time to take a break from modern medicine and just get back to basics.

We will show you how to make it through the most challenging situations and how to get the help you need. We will show you effective ways for coping with the stress you feel and turning to ancient remedies or more natural methods for getting pregnant.

It doesn't matter how long you have been trying or what kind of issues you have encountered, this book can help you through and make the process of getting pregnant seem much easier to deal with.

Though you may feel as if you are the only person going through this particular situation, it's important to know that you are not alone. There may be a number of reasons as to why conception is taking longer than anticipated and sometimes patience and time may be the best aid in the process. Fertility problems are on the rise due to a number of various environmental and lifestyle factors. Oftentimes there are no fertility issues at all, but rather the need to be patient and wait for conception to take place. Everything you feel in the process is normal and you must give yourself room to feel what you need to feel.

Coping With the Frustration

Since so many of us assume that it will just happen when we want to get pregnant, the notion of it taking some time and effort can be heartbreaking. For many women they spend their entire lives trying not to get pregnant.

Then when it comes time to wanting a baby and being ready for this next chapter, we naturally feel that it will happen on its own. So when that natural assumption is met with resistance and a much more concerted effort than we thought, it can throw us into a complete tailspin!

Frustration and Disappointment May Be a Very Normal Part of the Process

It is completely natural to feel frustrated with the process. The most normal and well-adjusted woman can have every emotion put to the test when she has problems getting pregnant.

It is the one thing in life that so many women want to experience— motherhood and the feeling of having our very own baby. . So when that is challenged or when we feel that this huge aspect of life may never happen, we feel disappointed, frustrated, and perhaps much much more.

It can often feel as though everybody around you is pregnant or having babies. When you are going through the process trying to get pregnant it can feel like you are alone and fighting against unseen forces. It can feel as though you are the only woman in the world without a baby and you just can't make sense of it.

The good news is, this is normal and that women around the world going through exactly the same thing mirror your thoughts. Most importantly, there's a good chance that absolutely nothing is wrong and it's just a matter of timing.

It is easy for people on the other side of pregnancy to say there's nothing to worry about, but when you are going through it, you do worry. You may have sleepless nights and you may even feel a bit detached for a while from friends and family. It's all-normal and you have to give yourself time to deal with your feelings.

This is where many women struggle and why it can make the process much more difficult. You need to give yourself time to grieve. Time to feel what you feel and then move forward so while many will tell you to move along and dismiss your feelings, which can actually be detrimental. Here we look at a few important things to remember as you struggle to cope at times.

Everything That You Feel is Normal

Start with this very important lesson and remember it—everything that you feel is normal! You are entitled to your feelings and there may be a lot of them that waiver from time to time.

Sometimes you may feel frustrated, other times you may feel depressed, then there's the anxiety, the anger, the bitter feelings, and you may at times feel hopeful and positive. The entire cycle, every single emotion within it, and the back and forth between the feelings is all-normal and all something you are entitled to!

Every woman who has had problems getting pregnant or wondered if it will ever happen for her has gone through what you are feeling. So if you have some bad days in the process… that's okay.

Don't beat yourself up or be mad at yourself for swinging from emotion to emotion. It's actually much healthier to let yourself feel those emotions than try to hide them.

You Are Truly Not Alone

When you are trying to get pregnant it can often feel like it is you against the world. You may even feel at odds with your spouse. Some days it will seem like everyone else is pregnant or has a baby, increasing your isolation.

If things are getting too tough, there are support groups available or your doctor can usually offer helpful insights and advice.

Many women find that once you relax and let yourself feel things, it can get easier. These days' fertility problems or even just having issues or time to get pregnant are very common.

We live in a fast paced world where we are achieving so much in a short space of time but pregnancy is not something we can schedule in and this is often a preconceived idea.

Summary:

There is a certain level of coping that must happen if a woman is struggling with her chances for conception. Though you may feel disillusioned, you are not alone and others have been in the same spot as you. Part of the process is to face your emotions head on so that you can move forward appropriately.

You are not alone, many others have been where you are and there is support available out there if you need it

Though you may need to try to adjust to everyday life, you also need to give yourself time to feel sad or angry or to cope with your emotions

Everything that you feel is normal and you should never feel bad about the emotions that you encounter along the way.

A Friend Gets Pregnant? It Is OK

It can feel like you just got hit with a truck—the moment you find out that one of your friends is pregnant! In normal circumstances you would be thrilled for them and be the first to help plan out their baby shower.

When you are on the other end of things and feeling like you are the only one not pregnant, it can be very difficult news to handle. You want to share in their joy but on a personal level you are grieving.

It's not to say that you are never going to have that moment in your own life, but realistically speaking it's just hard to be happy when it's not you. In that moment it can feel as if the entire world is against you, even though deep down you know that's not the case.

Nearly every woman who has struggled getting pregnant has had to deal with this situation. It's hard because you want to be happy for them but often your true emotions come out.

So how do you deal with this? How do you find happiness within you when all you feel is jealousy and sadness? It's not always easy but sometimes you just have to be happy for your friend when this situation comes about.

One important thing that nobody ever tells you is that it's okay to feel jealous. It's okay to feel bitter and angry and even frustrated that they are pregnant and not you. Feeling these emotions is part of coping and you need to give yourself some time and room to deal with it all. You just want to try your best not to show those emotions on the surface.

Here are some helpful tips to make this part of the process a bit more tolerable:

Offer your congratulations and try not to make it personal: They want to see you happy for them. Though they may recognize firsthand what is going on with you, they need you in that moment. Give yourself time to deal with your jealousy or emotions on your own and know that's okay—that it's actually healthy and normal! Beyond that though you need to be as upbeat as possible. At the very least offer your support and love, even if it's not easy for you. This will really be instrumental in helping you to get through the process!

Allow yourself some time to work through the emotions: You may feel frustrated, jealous, bitter, angry, and even depressed at their news. Feel what you need to feel. Deal with it on your own. The biggest thing to remember here is that you just don't want those emotions to overshadow your friend's joy.

Your time will come even if it doesn't feel that way: You are going to have a baby of your own someday and you must believe that! It may be next year or it may take longer than you anticipate. It could happen traditionally and you just need time or you may need to seek out fertility treatment. In this day and age there is almost always a way to give a woman a baby of her own, but you need to believe it will happen.

Have a conversation with your friend when the time is right. Be sure she knows how happy you are for her but you are going through your own personal issues. Don't make it about you but do be sure that she understands if you don't seem yourself. Sometimes a good open and honest dialogue can be so helpful and therapeutic for both parties so, if you can, invest the time in having this conversation.

If there are others who are negative or make you feel bad then learn to tune them out. It doesn't mean they are doing it on purpose; they can just be forgetful or insensitive. Forget the negative and be positive! You're bigger than that.

One of the hardest parts of going through fertility issues or a lengthy amount of time for conception is when somebody close to gets pregnant. Though you may feel like giving up or have a hard time adjusting to reality or even relating to that friend, you must show that life really does go on.

- You do need to function in normal life and remember that everybody has their turn.

- Allow yourself time to grieve on your own or away from your friend but do your best to be happy for them.

- Pay attention to your feelings and feel what you need to feel but do try to find a way to relate to your friend and remain close.

Knowing That You Are Not Alone

Start with the little things such as recognizing that you have not been told that you can't have children. You are not at the point yet where you have been told that there are fertility issues, and you may never get to that.

At this moment in time you are just having a hard time coping with the amount of time it's taking you to get pregnant. Know too that many women go through this and it is a very normal part of the process.

If you can recognize that many women have been through this and many more will in the future, that can be reassuring. You may find that on the roughest days you feel totally alone and isolated.

Rest assured though that other women have had the same struggles and are now proud mothers. Just as common as it is for it take awhile to get pregnant are the roller coaster of emotions that women go through in this situation.

Others Have Been Where You Are Right Now

So will it really make you feel better to know that others have struggled like you? Perhaps a bit if you know that this too shall pass. That's what you have to keep telling yourself and to recognize that you will get a baby somehow.

You will not go through this forever and there is help to be found. You may find it in the form of a supportive doctor, a friend that has been through the same thing, or even a support group.

To you six months may feel like six years but you have to do your best to gain perspective of the situation. Though it may feel like an eternity that you have been trying to get pregnant, it probably hasn't.

Though you may feel as though everybody around you is getting pregnant, they aren't. Though you may suspect that every mother you know got pregnant on her first try they truly didn't—and that's important to remember!

So the next time you are feeling low and alone and isolated, tell yourself that plenty of other women have been through this. Even those closest to you may have had their struggles and just don't advertise it.

It Hits Closer to Home Than You Realize

Upon further inspection you will find that women struggle with getting pregnant quite often, but it just might be on varying levels. This can offer some support and make your venture less stressful.

So as you try to remind yourself that you are not alone, there are a few things to keep in mind. These tips may really help to shed light on the problem and reassure you when you have doubts and frustrations.

Recognize that many women take awhile to get pregnant: Though some women may get pregnant as soon as they think about it, this is not the norm. These are the stories that people talk about because they are exceptions to the rule. Most women take at least a few months to get pregnant and that's the norm that nobody really speaks to. It takes awhile to get everything aligned and so you may just need to be patient with things and know that this happens to many women.

Know that the sentiments you feel are shared by many: The frustration, worry, anxiety, and even anger or sadness that you feel are all-normal. This is particularly true if a close friend or family member gets pregnant while you are trying. Don't beat yourself up over what you feel and now that it's all normal. Every woman who has taken awhile to get pregnant has had her struggles and her ups and downs. You are normal for feeling the things that you do, but just have to be careful not to act on it.

- ✓ Reach out if you need some reassurance: Talk to a trusted friend or family member, particularly if you know of one who went through a similar situation. Ask for help from your spouse, your parent, or a friend. Sometimes talking about it can be quite helpful and so you want to just get that reassuring talk to help you to feel more like yourself. If things get really difficult then by all means reach out for help in the form of a support group or other sponsored organization or activity. There is help for women in this situation so it's best to take advantage of it if you need it.

- ✓ Identify this as part of the process: If you are not somebody who got pregnant accidentally or unplanned, then this is all part of the process. The women who get pregnant right away don't recognize this process, as it's foreign to them. The truth is though that many of us struggle with this waiting game and it's therefore very normal. Wrap your head around the waiting aspect of getting pregnant and it can be a much smoother and more enjoyable journey for you.

Summary:

You truly are not alone and it's so important to remember that. Though you may feel as if you are the only one going through trouble in getting pregnant, many others have sat where you sit. It's crucial to keep this in mind and to recognize that your time will come, but also to get the support that you need if you find it a rough road to travel.

- ✓ There is support available to you in various forms if you find that you are having a hard time in coping with your conception issues

- ✓ Many others have gone through a similar process but may just not talk about it openly

- ✓ The feelings and the waiting period may all be part of a wonderful process

Talking to a Doctor and Getting A Thorough Assessment

Though many doctors will say that they don't even want to see you until you have been trying to get pregnant for a year, your instincts may tell you otherwise. If you are fearful or concerned about anything then this is a time to talk to your doctor and to see what exactly is going on. You are more than likely not at the point of full-fledged fertility testing, but you can at least get a clear picture of what is going on.

Many women find it wise to speak to their OBGYN at their annual appointment to discuss their current state. If you have been trying to get pregnant or are thinking about it, your annual appointment is a great time to discuss it. You may also wish to discuss any potential conditions or issues that could cause some problems down the road. In most instances the doctor will tell you that everything is just fine and to keep trying. What if that's not enough to ease your fears though?

Many women who have gone through this very situation will tell you that fertility is something that you have to take into your own hands. Some will say that they felt that they had to get a bit aggressive or at least proactive when it came to their desire to get pregnant. It's not that doctors aren't supportive but rather that they don't usually worry until it's been a significant amount of time in actively trying.

If you feel that you want to take matters into your own hands, then push for answers. Schedule an appointment with your OBGYN and take control over the appointment. To the woman going through difficulties in getting pregnant, even three short months may feel long enough to warrant concern. Most doctors will at least run a few basic tests just to be sure that everything is running smoothly with you. So take control over your fertility and put your mind at rest by getting into the doctor if you feel that's an important next step.

Make Your Appointment Really Count

When you do get in with the doctor you want this appointment to really help matters. This is an appointment that you may need to be proactive with, but it should really help to calm your fears. You may not be sure of what is in store for you, but this is a great way to move forward with a clear head and a clean bill of health. If there were to be something amiss or some medical condition present, then this is the time that you want to become aware of that.

So think through a few fundamental aspects of that first appointment and go in prepared. Consider the following to help you along the way:

- ✓ Go in with a lot of questions: You can and should use this forum to ask a great deal of questions. Go in with an entire list asking about everything from your cycle to your periods themselves to the best time to try. Talk about the experience that you have been having and walk them through your process thus far. It may just be that you are trying too early or too late and so this is a great time to get everything flushed out.

- ✓ Ask what you can do to help track things properly: For some women it may not be enough to just track the days of their period on a calendar. You may be somebody who really needs to know clearly when you ovulate as it isn't clear. Discuss with your doctor what methods work best and which tools they want you to use. Getting a medical opinion on this factor rather than relying on what your friends may have done can really help to shed light on things.

✓ Discuss any fears that you may have: If you have a good relationship with your doctor then talk about anything that you may fear. This can be a great form of emotional support coming from a trusted expert. This is also a good time to ensure that your doctor is the right one moving forward, as they should be there to help now and throughout your pregnancy.

✓ Ensure that you get a full exam and any extra testing that you may be interested in: You should automatically get a full exam but you may need to push for any testing beyond that. If you are worried about your hormone levels or if ovulation is actually taking place then ask what can be done to assess. Your doctor may not offer this readily and so you may need to go in as an educated consumer. You want to rule anything out at the beginning and if you get the proper blood work and exam done then you can really rest assured that everything is just fine.

Natural Remedies to Increase Your Chances

A healthy lifestyle is a big part of increasing your chances of getting pregnant, but you can take things further than that. If you want to go for the more natural route then there are plenty of solutions and products out there that can help. You do need to be careful to read labels and to ensure that you don't fall for a product that offers more than it can really offer. When in doubt, talk to your doctor so that you have all of the facts because this can save you a lot of aggravation and money.

That being said, there are some solutions that can work quite well. These are mostly driven by natural herbs and even vitamins and minerals, which can offer some complementary medical support. These can help to prepare the body for pregnancy more effectively and have been used for ages to assist in this manner. If something is lacking within your body or if perhaps it's not properly prepared then these natural remedies can help to fill in the gaps.

Do be careful to ensure that you get the most natural forms of these herbs and remedies as possible. Try not to be drawn into mixtures as the more natural the product the more that it's going to help you. Amongst the top choices of the natural remedies are a few that offer health benefits, but more importantly help to boost chances of conception. They work differently but they ultimately help to prepare a woman's body for pregnancy and therefore increase the likelihood that the environment is ready to accept conception.

The best of the natural remedies include the following:

✓ **Green Tea:** The great thing about green tea in general is that it offers assistance with repairing any damage done within the body. The damage that may come about due to toxins that we consume or ingest can often interfere with the ability to conceive. Green tea offers antioxidant powers and goes after any toxins or related damage done to the body. This may be just what you need to get a jump-start on conception and therefore why this natural remedy may be for you. Try green tea extract as a natural herb. Try also drinking a couple of cups of green tea each day as it offers a slight amount of caffeine which is effective when you are trying to cut down on it but still need a healthy boost.

✓ **Red Raspberry Leaf:** This is about as powerful as you can get when it comes to natural remedies and therefore highly recommended as a solution. Red raspberry leaf helps to tone the uterus and the pelvic region in general. It has been recognized as a way of naturally boosting fertility for centuries and so it is finally being recognized within the mainstream. You may find that you get the most out of this herb when you partner it with peppermint, and so this combination can be a woman's best friend when it comes to problems with conception.

✓ **Ladies Mantle:** This is known as a sort of tonic that helps dramatically with conception. This not only helps to strengthen the uterus, but it can help with the monthly cycle as well. Women may turn to this if they are having irregular monthly cycles or are just trying to get things on track. So this is an excellent herb to help with all of the related fertility issues as it provides support overall.

✓ **Red Clover:** This remedy helps to restore and balance the hormonal function and nourishes the uterus all at the same time. In addition, red clover also promotes estrogen production, which can be a problem in some women. In addition to containing estrogen like compounds, red clover also helps to relax the nervous system and promote conception simultaneously. This is an herb that you definitely want to look into for when given in proper doses it really does offer tremendous help with conception.

It's best to go to a natural health store to find these herbs and figure out what sort of dosage and combination makes sense for you. These herbs may be taken together but it's always best to get medical advice and to take into consideration your particular situation. If nothing else these may help to properly and naturally prepare the body for conception without any harmful side effects.

These are a great step to consider before moving into fertility treatments or more extreme measures. You also want to be sure that in addition to clean and healthy living, that vitamins and minerals are part of your repertoire. They often contain compounds and even antioxidants that may help to get the body into the best shape possible for conception to occur.

The Power of Acupuncture

There are certain solutions within conception that have been around for centuries that have somehow not quite made it into the mainstream. One such solution is acupuncture and though it is becoming more common, many doctors don't necessarily understand or promote it. This is the type of service that you usually have to look into through a complementary or alternative type of treatment facility, but it may be worth your effort.

Many people have a tendency to turn their noses up at acupuncture, usually because they don't understand it. Others are fearful of needles and therefore discount this helpful service due to their fear. Another issue that faces acupuncture is that it simply isn't recognized by the medical community as a whole for the helpful solution that it may be. If you happen to find a doctor or a facility that supports or offers this, then you are heading in the right direction.

Understanding How It Actually Works

The way that acupunctures works is that needles are placed strategically in the body for whatever may be ailing you. There is a belief that is centuries old that there are various regions within the body and they can become closed, clogged, or even shut down. When this happens you end up with illness or health problems overall, and there are so many different symptoms that this may show up through.

So when it comes to fertility specifically the belief is that the region in the body that affects this may become closed off and therefore conception becomes impossible. Acupuncture goes to work to help "unblock" these regions and allow conception to occur. Though this may sound unusual or not the conventional school of thought or treatment, it has been around for years and is a widely accepted part of Eastern medicine and culture.

Depending on the specific fertility issues or what the woman may be going through, this dictates where the needles are placed. It all depends on if the woman suffers from irregular monthly cycles, an actual condition like endometriosis, or is just having problems in getting pregnant overall. Small needles are placed atop the skin in a very noninvasive manner to help concentrate the efforts on this region of the body.

After the needles are inserted, usually very quickly and painlessly, a light is placed on this region and the woman rests comfortably for almost an hour. Though this may sound anything but relaxing, it is often found to be a source of comfort for the woman going through it. Though it does require some getting used to, this can be an amazing treatment and has been found to be highly effective for women who turn to it.

Considering a Helpful and Out of the Box Solution

Though many doctors won't necessarily promote acupuncture, there is no doubting the power that it has. This is a practice that has been used for centuries and is a recognized aspect of Eastern medicine. The women who try acupuncture find it if nothing else to be an excellent stress relief and report feeling almost weightless as they lay there to relax. The needles go to work to help "unblock" the regions of the body that control fertility and the woman gets to enjoy a great relief from stress as this happens.

This is well worth looking into for a woman who is open minded and who wants to try everything before she turns to the more accepted fertility treatments abroad. Though this is often not covered by insurance, it is a treatment well worth trying if a woman is struggling with conception. There is nothing to lose and the potential for everything to gain, but it's important to go in with an open mind and an ability to relax and let this ancient treatment work for you.

Acupuncture has been working for centuries for fertility issues and for health problems overall and so it's an excellent natural remedy to consider in your quest towards conception. Sometimes you need to think outside of the box, and this is one of those instances, which may really work for you in the end!

Reduce Your Stress

You are going to hear it more times than you care to admit in the process of trying to get pregnant—don't be so stressed out and just relax! Though this can make for some rather annoying and repetitive advice, there is some merit to it. Well worth mentioning though that this can often be easier said than done when you are going through the process and you feel overwhelmed and the stress is at a maximum.

The truth is that there are some great ways to relax but it may be slightly different for everyone. You need to get in touch with what allows you to relax whether it's yoga, deep breathing, some time alone, or even a pedicure with a trusted friend. There is something that we all rely upon to help us relax and feel centered, and when it comes to conception you are going to need this.

The more that you can allow yourself to relax, the better your chances of conception will be. That's a very powerful concept but it's all too easy to get caught up in the small details of what you are feeling and experiencing and allow that to rule your life. Stress seems inevitable and so it basically becomes a matter of managing what causing you stress within your life. Though those that mean well will tell you to take it easy and to learn to relax, sometimes that may seem almost impossible.

Not only can learning to manage your stress now help you to get pregnant, but it can benefit you throughout your pregnancy and new role as well. Getting your body to relax and slowing down what goes on in your mind is a great habit to get into, so embrace it now. There are always going to be areas of stress in our life, but it's all in how we handle it that gives it power or makes it easier to dismiss. The less that you let stress take a hold of your health and your life, the more that you will benefit from this for conception and even beyond!

Why Stress Management Really Matters

Learning to manage your stress matters in every area of your life, but especially with conception. If you can learn to master this often challenging and frustrating aspect of your life then you can reap some amazing rewards—and get to have that baby that you've always dreamed of much faster!

Confront your sources of stress and don't let them take power over you: Recognizing that we all have areas of stress in our lives, it's important to come to terms with them. If you can define what causes you stress then you can learn to take control over them much more effectively. Though these sources of stress may still exist, you can learn to manage them before they get the best of you. Sure this takes some diligence and dedication, but it makes for a much healthier way of living. You have the power to choose how you let stressful areas of life affect you and it's time to manage it once and for all.

Know that reducing your stress can help to increase your chances of conception: If you can wrap your mind around this concept then your fertility is going to benefit as a result. Learning to manage your stress can really truly improve your chances of getting pregnant. Stress can have a direct impact upon your monthly cycles, your regularity, and even your ovulation. When you can take a deep breath, gain perspective, and relax then you start to get to more normalcy. This usually makes for a more regular cycle and therefore increases your chances for conception in the process.

Recognize that stress is bad for your physical, mental, and emotional health: Stress isn't good for you overall and it's time to recognize that. Stress can play into health conditions in your physical condition and cause you to feel fatigued, lack focus, or even get sick more easily. Stress can make you feel worn down, depressed, and really cause some short and long term health conditions. So knowing that it's time to take control over the areas that cause you stress, not only as it pertains to fertility but to your health as a whole. The sooner that you learn this the more that you contribute to better physical, mental, and emotional health in the here and now and well beyond.

Creating a Healthy Lifestyle

A healthy lifestyle is good for so many reasons and yet so few of us actually participate in one. Though we may have good intentions there is bound to be at least one area of our lives that we can improve upon. This is good for the overall big picture of health but it also plays into fertility and most of us don't recognize or realize that. If you can get yourself into the very best picture of health then you are getting your body ready for conception sooner.

So some of these elements may impact your conception chances directly and some indirectly. It's best to get rid of the bad habits now and prepare yourself for clean and healthy living, as that will become crucial during pregnancy and beyond. The sooner that you can adapt to these components the better and the more that you will gain these benefits. However many people find that they are questioning what exactly makes up a healthy lifestyle and so it may be worth reviewing.

Here we take a look at what makes up a healthy lifestyle, and more importantly how you can get this to work for you. Many people notice almost instantly how much better they feel and even look. Along with the other health benefits if you follow these guidelines you are taking natural steps and methods to get yourself to a healthy weight range, which is another important factor for preparing the body for conception and pregnancy

Eating the Right Foods in the Right Manner

There is great power in food and we don't tend to think of that. Rather than grabbing processed foods on the go, try to be mindful of what you are eating and prepare your food accordingly. When you eat processed foods you are taking in far too many additives, preservatives, and sodium which may act as toxins within the body and cause harm.

So it's clear that eating a proper diet made up of each of the food groups on the food pyramid is the way to go. This means that you should focus on lean proteins, low fat dairy products, whole grains, good fats, and plenty of fresh fruits and vegetables. These foods will offer vitamins, minerals, antioxidants, and fiber that the body needs to sustain itself and to stay strong and vital. This is the way to eat to lose weight, to get the most out of your food, and to generally feel better towards conception and to life in general.

You also need to be mindful of the way in which you eat your foods too. You should be eating smaller meals more frequently throughout the day. This keeps your energy levels up and ensures that you aren't tempted to give in to nutritionally void foods. Try to aim for 5-6 mini meals each day. To get the most out of each mini meal try to combine food groups whenever possible as you get the most value out of each and every bite. Carefully plan out your meals each week and prepare them each day to ensure that you are eating in the best way possible.

Learning to Embrace Truly Challenging Exercise

Fitness is an important part of weight loss, but are there other health benefits beyond that? Many experts are finding that fitness before pregnancy can help to get the body ready for not only carrying a baby but bouncing back faster after baby is born. When you challenge yourself in your fitness regimen you tend to shed fat, burn calories, and build muscle tone in the process.

The fitness regimen that you take on should include a combination of cardio and strength training exercises. This will help you to lose weight and get to your best shape yet. This truly can help with conception and will allow you to manage your stress better as well. You will learn to love exercise during this stage of your life and may very well be able to enjoy it during pregnancy as well.

Getting Plenty of Rest

In addition to managing your stress you want to learn to get plenty of rest in the process. Our body needs the optimal eight hours of sleep each night to rebuild, repair, and regain energy. So though you may have far too much to do in a day, when you shortchange yourself on sleep you are only hurting yourself. You feel less focused, lack energy, and may get sick more often when you aren't well rested.

Though there may be more of an indirect link between getting enough rest and conception, it's a concept worth considering. You are at your best when you get the optimal eight hours of sleep each night and so you should be aiming for it. This is part of a truly healthy lifestyle and allows the other components to work appropriately if you make this a priority.

Taking Good Care of Yourself

Quit smoking, drinking excessive caffeine or alcohol, and kick all of the bad habits. This will get you ready for pregnancy and really allow you to feel your best. Getting the toxins such as these out of your body may truly help conception directly and ensure that you are in the best possible shape for pregnancy. Though the bad habits may have ruled your life up until now, it's time to take control over them once and for all.

In addition to managing your stress you want to really make the effort to take good care of yourself. This may mean that you make yourself a priority. It may mean that you get rid of negative outside influences and learn to embrace the positive ones.

This may mean that you shift your mindset and start to focus on the true power of positive thinking. Whatever you can do to make yourself a priority and truly take care of yourself will contribute to better health. This in turn increases your chances of conception and ensures that you are the best that you can possibly be now and when you do get pregnant!

The Power of Positive Thinking and Attitude In Your Quest

Along with the stress reduction that you will hear so much about is adapting to the right attitude. Many will argue that it's easier said than done which is true. The reality however is that if you can somehow use positive thinking to power you through your journey it's going to make things much easier. Not only do you have the right mindset to help you in coping with anything, but you also have a much better way of handling any obstacles that may come your way as well.

The reality is that a positive mindset may be what makes the difference between struggling in your journey and making it through with flying colors. You are going to have days of sheer frustration. You are going to second guess yourself and you are going to feel overwhelmed, full of anxiety, and overall stressed out with the circumstance that you are in. What's important to remember in all of this is that you can master these elements much more easily if you can remain calm, positive, and have the right attitude.

No matter what you have to believe that this is all going to work out. You have to believe and even envision that you are holding a baby of your own someday. You have to know that with whatever negative circumstances may come your way you can overcome them and stay strong. True strength comes from the ability to cast aside your fears and focus on what it really takes to make it through this sometimes-challenging time. Though you may feel tempted to give in to what is causing you stress, that will only hurt you in the end.

If you can understand and stand behind the power of positive thinking you are going to have a much easier time of things in general. You will realize that the right attitude can really and truly make a difference in your life, for your conception journey and beyond. Some will say that positive thinking really and truly can make the differences. Others will tell you that it will just make things easier along the way. No matter what you should never underestimate the power of positive thinking as it can help you in a number of different ways and so it's well worth focusing on when it comes to your conception journey. So let's see just how positive thinking and the right attitude can help you along the way.

The Power of the Mind and the Right Attitude

Never feel that positive thinking is just a nicety. For when you truly invest in this, particularly as it relates to your conception journey, you start to really reap the rewards. Here are some fundamental ways that the right attitude and positive mindset can really help you along the way:

The journey is much easier to take on if you have a positive attitude to make it through: When you think and feel positive there is no stopping you. There is great strength in all that you do and you are better equipped to deal with things in life. When it comes to your ability to get pregnant a negative attitude can go hand in hand with stress. So when you feel stressed or you are overcome with anxiety you are much more likely to create a less than ideal condition for getting pregnant. The more that you can be positive and stay that way the more likely you are to be calm. In the end that ultimately means that positivity will equate to the right environment for conception to take place. This really does work and it makes you feel better in the process!

You are much more likely to be successful if you let the right mindset guide you: Not only does positivity help you to remain calm but it can create that "can do" attitude. When you invest in yourself through positive thinking you start to see the finish line. In the end this means that you are focused on and envisioning what you ultimately want to happen. Visualization is a major component of the right mindset and therefore really helps you to stay true to what you want. It's close to you, it's within reach, and the positive mindset really helps to guide you towards your goal. You can consider this to be an important part of a healthy lifestyle and therefore stay focused on what you want to become yours.

Consider the fundamentals of the Law of Attraction: Whether you are truly invested in it or not there is the philosophy within this Law that says the universe will give you what you put out to it. Meaning that if you are positive, strong, and focused on your goals you will get what you are after. If you put positive energy out to the universe that is what it will return. This Law, goal setting, and the power of positive thinking and a strong mental attitude are all what will help you to achieve what you want. This is very powerful and therefore you start to really feel strong and believe that a baby will be yours. It is at that moment that the stress dissipates, the inner strength takes over, and you are surrounded by nothing but positive sentiments. So whatever you believe now, reevaluate just how important the mind is within this and therefore turning to a positive mental journey really is worth the investment!

Learning To Adapt to Real Life Settings Involving Babies...When All You Want Is One Of Your Own!

It can truly feel like a dagger when it happens—that moment that you see a friend or family member holding their newborn baby! It's not that you aren't happy for them; it's just that you aren't in a place to feel nothing but pure happiness for them. This is a common sentiment felt by women in this situation and therefore it is well worth considering and preparing for in the best way that you can. Real life situations like these will likely replay over and over again, and all you can do is be ready for them when they occur.

It's not that you're a selfish person; it's just that sometimes it's rather difficult to cope with these situations. When all you want is a baby and that's all that you can focus on and visualize then it's truly difficult to feel blissful for somebody else when it happens. So how do you handle these situations that are bound to play out over and over again? How do you stay strong in front of those that are enjoying a pregnancy or new baby when all you feel is sad and jealous?

It's all about adaptation and being prepared, as those are the two elements that will help you through. You now know what tools you need to make it through the journey and this is one part of it. If you can adapt to real life settings and try to mentally prepare yourself then it will make life in general much easier and more enjoyable. It's not to say that it will always be easy and it's not as if you can ignore your feelings, but this is a great way of making it through your own personal journey in a much more effective way.

You need to find the strength within yourself to get started and then continue to get in touch with it to move on with your life. These are the scenarios that tend to play over and over again for anybody in your situation and so the sooner that you can learn to stay ahead of them; the better your life will be as you move forward.

Learning to Stay On Top of Things

These situations are always going to be a part of life so in the end it's all in how you deal with them. Here are some fundamental and helpful things to keep in mind as you move along:

Recognize that life will go on and you have to go on with it: You can't control what goes on in others lives. You can't manage when others will have babies or how it will all transpire. The only thing that you can manage is how you react to things. Life will go on, loved ones close to you will get pregnant and have babies, and so you have to roll with it. You have to find a place of inner strength within you to help guide you through the tough times and allow you to rise above what you may be feeling inside. This is all part of the process and what will help you to cope accordingly.

Prepare yourself mentally and try to stay strong: Though it may be hard for you it's important to find and use your inner strength. You want to use your best mental attitude to help you through the difficult circumstances such as seeing a friend's newborn for the first time. Positive attitude and mindset are all a part of this and so the more in tune that you can be to this; the better off you will be in the end. Being mentally prepared and strong is ultimately what will help you through the tough times.

Don't let these situations overwhelm you, do your best to take control over them: You can control your emotions and reactions, and that's important to remember. You must be the person that stays strong on the outside and shows happiness for those closest to you. Remember that you will have your turn and hold your own baby but for now it's important to stay strong and control your emotional reaction. Positive thinking, inner strength, and the right mindset are all going to be what helps you through those sometimes difficult days so use this to power you through and it will really keep you strong and overall happy for others and for the future that awaits you!

Doing Your Best To Let Nature Take Its Course

It's not enough to say that you need to take the stress out of things, as you actually have to live that. It's not enough to say that you need to stay positive and not let things overwhelm you as you must do it. The reality is that saying that you are going to do the right things is one thing, but actually doing them is quite another. So while you may be focused in on moving forward with the best of intentions, you must actually make the necessary changes if you want to reap the rewards.

To move forward in great harmony and to ultimately get to conception you must stay focused on living the advice that you see here. The tips provided within this book come from expertise and a place of knowing that you must take stress and negativity out of the equation. That's often easier said than done but these changes will ultimately be what makes the difference for your ability to conceive or not. So it's all about taking this advice and then applying it to your everyday life.

So as you think about how to get rid of the negative and embrace the positive it's all about letting things happened in the way that they were intended. Though you may be saying that you believe it will happen on the outside you have to actually know it and live it on the inside. You can't pretend when it comes to these things as that won't work. In many instances therefore that may mean that you need to let things go and relax a bit. Again when you are going through this, it's not always as easy as all of that but its well worth it and essential if you wish to get pregnant.

One major component of this in your world is to let go of some of the science. You can drive yourself crazy thinking about when you ovulated or when you will be ready for conception. You can go mad thinking about your cycle and relating it to the right time to try for a baby. The reality is that you can control some factors but not all of them. Therefore sometimes you have to let go a little bit. Sometimes you need to just let nature take its course and let the right things fall into place. So as you consider what it takes to move forward in the best manner, you need to learn to sit back, relax, and wait for the magic to happen so to speak.

Applying What You Have Learned in Your Life

So as you think of an effective strategy moving forward you need to really allow things to happen without trying to control them. This takes some practice and diligence but in the end it allows things to work out much more cohesively. Here are some great ways to let things happen without giving in to excessive anxiety:

Take the science out of things for a while: Put aside the thermometers, the ovulation tests, the pregnancy tests, and any other tools that you've been using. Sometimes these can really add stress to the process and unnecessarily. You will start to get an idea of what your body is doing and how your cycle works as you move forward anyhow. So get rid of the science at least for now and just get back to basics. Share time with your spouse and when you take the science out of things it can actually be much more enjoyable in the process.

Use your new positive attitude to really help guide you along the way: As you get back to basics start to adapt to a more positive version of you. The positive attitude and mindset that you adapt to is what will truly help to guide you through. This is far more effective than any other tool and yet allows you to take the stress out of the process. Stop worrying about what day it is in your cycle or what's going on with you or others and instead be guided by your new philosophy and positive attitude for more effectiveness in the process.

Go back to basics and enjoy this time with your significant other: When you do get pregnant your relationship goes through an adjustment period. It's all worth it in the end but just for now enjoy some time with your loved one. This is the last time it will be just the two of you and so take advantage of that and embrace who you are as a couple. Sometimes this can take the stress out of things and help to prepare you in an entirely different way. You will really learn to fall in love all over again and learn to appreciate this person you are with, rather than just looking at them as the man who will help you to create a child. This is a great way to move forward and to do so in great harmony!

Discussing and Considering Next Steps in Your Journey

Though it's always best to work through each of the steps to help you along to conception, sometimes it may be necessary to consider next steps. If you have been trying for a while or if you fear that something just isn't right then it may be time to progress with asking for help. If nothing else you want to be diligent about trusting your instincts and moving forward with alternative steps if you feel that they are necessary.

Suffice it to say that there are many times when a woman fears that something is wrong when in actuality it really isn't. Many women feel that pregnancy isn't happening fast enough and therefore march into their doctor's office, many times prematurely. There's nothing wrong with this and doctors are certainly used to it, but it may be wise to wait it out a bit and try all of the other steps outlined in this book. If however you really think that something is wrong, know that you are not the only woman who has gone rushing into her doctor's office for some sound medical advice.

In most instances it will be found that there is absolutely nothing wrong and it's a matter of timing. Many women are premature to worry and to seek out medical advice, but it may be that they need to hear it from a trained professional. Some women may fear that their cycle is too irregular or that they aren't having intercourse on the appropriate days. If it's a matter of education then try to handle matters on your own. If however you are truly concerned or something seems wrong, then trust your instincts and take matters into your own hands.

If you are truly concerned and want to seek out help in the process or consider next steps, then consider the following tips, which may prove to be quite helpful:

Always trust your instincts: You know yourself and the process better than anybody else. If your cycle is off or if things just seem different within your own body then go with your gut. Your instincts may be the best predictor if something truly is wrong, but know that sometimes we have a tendency to get ahead of ourselves. You should always trust your instincts when it comes to health issues, as it's better to be safe than sorry. Do however be sure that you have exhausted all other options, tried the tactics recommended here, and are truly at a loss as to why pregnancy isn't occurring. Know too that many doctors won't even want to talk to you until you have been trying diligently for about a year.

Know when it's time to ask for a bit of help: Be your own advocate and move things along if you feel that it's necessary. Though you may recognize that it hasn't been that long or that you are on top of when ovulation is occurring or adapting to a truly healthy lifestyle, you may just need some medical insight. A doctor is well versed in dealing with conception issues. They may ask for some tests to be run for you or your partner, which if nothing else can help to ease your mind. Sometimes it's just something like that, which can springboard you into the settled feeling and the realization that pregnancy will occur and that it's just a matter of when. You may wish to make an appointment with your doctor if you've been trying for a while, if you fear that something is just wrong within your cycle or your body, or when you feel that you've exhausted all of your resources and just need some help.

Consider all of your options: One of the first things that most doctors will want to do if you go to see them is to run some blood work. Ask for help in detecting that ovulation is in fact occurring. Ask for tests to be run for both you and your partner, as the issue may not just be on your side of things. Ask for what your options will be in terms of exploratory work before you would ever move forward. Before you agree to any fertility medication or treatments, make sure that you are aware of and in tune with all of the options that lie before you. Ask the tough questions, be sure that you understand your specific situation, and then use this information to guide you forward in the most appropriate path for your specific situation. You can make educated decisions and ensure that the right things happen which will ultimately result in pregnancy, but sometimes you need to know when it's time to take matters into your own hands!

The Final Word

You are not the first or the last woman to face the difficulties in getting pregnant. That's an important note and so you want to really let that sink in. Though getting pregnant can be a much more challenging and difficult process than many anticipate, the reality is that it will happen for most women in the most natural way possible. Though many have been through this process in a similar manner, those that go through it tend to feel alone.

There are certain realities to the process of conception, and some of them involve the world around you. It's important to come to terms with what is going on within you but not to let it rule your life. Though it may take you longer than anticipated, it will more than likely happen and you will soon be able to enjoy a baby of your own. You do need to recognize that actually getting pregnant is a much more involved process than most realize.

There are great ways to help prepare your body for pregnancy. We have looked what you can do within your own lifestyle and your own body to help things along. We have looked at how you can move throughout your days and handle everyday scenarios to ensure that you can handle the journey to conception. It's not always easy but it's well worth it if in the end you are holding your own little bundle of joy. It may be a matter of learning how to cope with things and how to function properly when conception becomes more involved than you realized.

You can make healthy changes within yourself to help the process along. You can work towards making a transition that will better your life and improve your chances for conception. Though the road may be long and sometimes challenging, you can learn to make effective change within yourself now that will increase your odds and make you a much happier person in the process. The changes that you make now will help your life in general and ensure that you get to really enjoy pregnancy and motherhood in the end.

So while conception may take a little while and may be more involved than you had anticipated, now you know what to expect and how to handle it. The steps that you take now and the advice that you apply to your own life can make all the difference. Cast aside all of the negativity and outside influences and focus on what really matters in the end. You now have all the tools, tips, and advice that you need to make a difference in your conception journey. It's time to move forward on a positive note and to enjoy what lies ahead—a baby will be yours and now it's time to embrace the journey every step of the way!

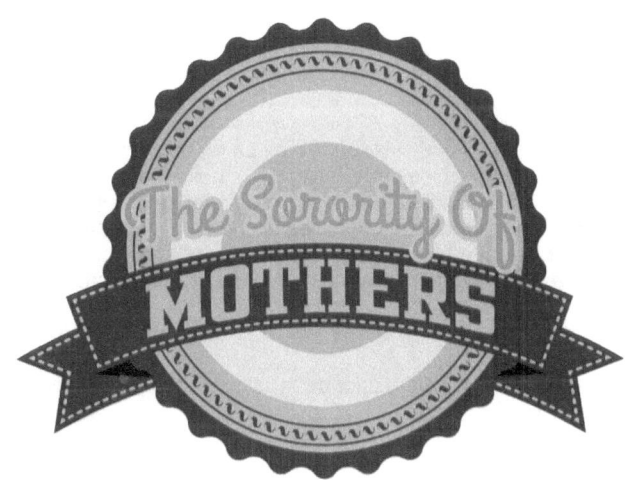

Copyright © 2014

Disclaimer

Legal Notice: - The author and publisher of this book and the accompanying materials have used their best efforts in preparing the material. The author and publisher make no representation or warranties with respect to the accuracy, applicability, fitness or completeness of the contents of this book. The information contained in this book is strictly for educational purposes. Therefore, if you wish to apply ideas contained in this book, you are taking full responsibility for your actions.

The author and publisher disclaim any warranties (express or implied), merchantability, or fitness for any particular purpose. The author and publisher shall in no event be held liable to any party for any direct, indirect, punitive, special, incidental or other consequential damages arising directly or indirectly from any use of this material, which is provided "as is", and without warranties.

As always, the advice of a competent legal, tax, accounting or other professional should be sought. The author and publisher do not warrant the performance, effectiveness or applicability of any sites listed or linked to in this book. All links are for information purposes only and are not warranted for content, accuracy or any other implied or explicit purpose.